MOVE

MOVE

Get Inspired For Your Health

CHERYL FISCUS JENKINS

authorHOUSE®

AuthorHouse™ LLC
1663 Liberty Drive
Bloomington, IN 47403
www.authorhouse.com
Phone: 1-800-839-8640

Published by AuthorHouse   09/13/2013

ISBN: 978-1-4918-1979-1 (sc)
ISBN: 978-1-4918-1978-4 (e)

Library of Congress Control Number: 2013916882

LIABILITY DISCLAIMER

CONTENTS

DEDICATION

This book would never have been possible without answered prayers in bringing it to life. A special thanks to my fitness class students who have inspired me throughout the years with their faithfulness and energy and to all of the people striving every day to improve their health. To my husband for putting up with my late nights at the gym and to my niece, Alex, for her prudent editing of this book.

INTRODUCTION

Let me take you back 32 years when I was silenced to a sedentary state due to the pain and stiffness of rheumatoid arthritis.

In one week, I transformed from being a lively, athletic and energetic teen-ager to lying on the couch barely able to move.

I moved whatever body parts I could from a resting position. Forced myself to stand up when my knees screamed to sit back down. Raised my arms when my shoulders insisted the place for them was hanging by my side.

Being sedentary was by far the most painful part in dealing with my illness because for years I had been active in recreational sports and as a gymnast and cheerleader. Even in those difficult times the drive to stay active never left my mind.

Staying physically fit became an emotional driver for me as I worked through the suffering associated with new onset and uncontrolled RA. I would have done just about anything in the early stages of my illness to move forward from the pain and stiffness of being bedridden for days.

So when I decided to write this book for beginning exercisers after almost three decades of teaching aerobics at various fitness facilities, most people thought I would write specifically for those with arthritis.

I love teaching individuals with arthritis who endure the same symptoms I have dealt with in my years of facing this chronic disease. The movement can have such a profound impact on their overall health and well-being.

Before beginning this book, though, another group of individuals weighed even more heavily on my heart and mind. Those thoughts stemmed from my journalism days years ago when I wrote for the local newspaper about health and wellness.

On a chilly spring morning this year, I pulled out an old newspaper clipping of mine dated February 9, 1997. The bold case headline read, "How Healthy Are We?"

This story unfolded seven months after the well-known study Physical Activity and Health: A Report of the Surgeon General was released in July 1996 and prepared by the CDC. The report fascinated me as it assessed the role physical activity, performed most days of the week, played in preventing disease and in maintaining a high quality of life. It also shouted a call to action about the hazards of being sedentary, and that physical inactivity was a serious nationwide problem.

I assumed most people were active until I read this report and realized I needed to a better job as a health and fitness writer to spread the word about the effects of sedentary lifestyles. I never would have imagined my journalism days would come full circle so many years later and bring me right back here writing a book about the need for more physical activity.

The "How Healthy Are We?" article gave the national Surgeon General's report a local Columbus, Ind., focus with an overall assessment and study of its health status. My hometown fared well in some categories but failed to make the grade in two very important aspects: weight and physical activity.

I remember the story well because it was one of my last before transitioning careers from full-time writing to full-time healthcare. The words provided a deep public health message and brought to light important facts that could have made a difference in someone's well-being.

Today I read newspaper articles all of the time about the effects and prevalence of obesity and sedentary lifestyles in the United States, and particularly, in my home state of Indiana. The articles make me flashback to my early days of RA when the disease caused a temporary, but difficult, sedentary setback in my otherwise active and healthy life.

My goal with this book is that no one be left behind in this very important message regarding physical activity and the many ways it can help improve one's health in certain situations. I am calling all non-exercisers who have been told they should exercise or know they should or those who simply want to give it a try to step forward for improved health.

At this point in my fitness career, I want to bridge the gap between health and healthcare and to use my illness as an example of how important it is to take interest in your well-being and to take care of yourself to the best of your ability.

I want you to start this journey now by scheduling an appointment with your doctor for the OK to become more physically active. Ask questions and get details on what you can and cannot do in relation to your specific health conditions.

MOVE: Get Inspired For Your Health is a navigational tool to move you in the right direction toward a more active lifestyle. The book has been years in the making and is my life story of how movement has kept me strong and healthy, even at my weakest moments.

I have been inspired by all of the people around me whose health and mobility have become so important they take the time and make the effort to sweat their way into better shape every week, every month, year after year. This year, I hope it is time for you to get inspired, too, as we move through this fitness journey together.

Chapter One
MY INSPIRATION

The day of the eighth-grade basketball tournament, my feet were swollen three times their size and every joint in my body throbbed with even the smallest movement. Tears filled my eyes as I forced on my cheerleading saddle shoes before the game early that morning and performed splits and jumps throughout the day.

Not yet diagnosed with rheumatoid arthritis and unprepared to deal with the pain, I thought this day would never end.

My friends and I had a slumber party that Friday night before, excited to participate in the annual Columbus, Ind., junior high school basketball tournament on Saturday. We stayed up most of the night, as teen-age girls do, laughing, talking and playing with hairstyles for the next day.

It was a welcome break from the sickness I had felt for two weeks prior to the weekend events with pain and stiffness in most joints, slight swelling, limited range of motion and extreme fatigue.

I was the smallest on the cheerleading squad, always on top of pyramids or doing flips out front and landing in the splits. That athleticism came easily until January 1982 when even little things, such as turning on the shower, sent a shock of pain from my wrist up my arm. Gone were the days when I could climb effortlessly up the pyramid, pose for a moment then dismount to the hardwood floor.

On this Saturday AM, after about two hours of sleep, it took everything in me to put my feet to the floor and stand up from the bed without falling down. The smile I typically wore was filled with worry about what was going on with my joints and whether I could struggle through school activities that day.

When the buzzer sounded at the end of the first half, I held back tears from the pain I had endured that morning and the relief of it being partially over. Could I possibly continue as our squad practiced and prepped for the last two basketball quarters?

Unwilling to admit defeat, inform my parents what was going on and go home to rest, I pulled myself together for round two. Stubbornness had kicked in, and I would pay for it later.

Cheering the second half of that basketball game shaped my purpose and drive for many years to come as I have faced the headaches of chronic illness. It is the backbone of why I am writing this book today to inspire you toward improved health.

The longer I cheered and jumped and kicked and performed splits in the gymnasium that day, the better I felt.

Though distressed by some discomfort, my smile came back slightly, and my joints moved more freely. The tears I shed that night were those of end of basketball season emotions not of my inability and frustration to do what had always come so easily.

There is no question I overdid it that Saturday—almost to the point of stupidity. The muscle and joint pain I endured Sunday and many days following were ten-fold worse than while cheering the team's last game.

The following week, my knees buckled with stiffness and pain every step I walked into my future with RA. The diagnosis that following Friday, after doctors' appointments and many medical tests, rocked my world at age 14.

On Sunday AM, it took me 20 minutes to sit up in bed and another 30 minutes to walk from my room and down one flight of stairs for breakfast. I actually gave up on walking 25 minutes in, sat down on the steps and scooted the rest of the way to the living room.

With my feet again the size of grapefruits and every joint in my body piercing with pain, it would have been easy that morning (and sometimes months and years later) to throw in the towel to rheumatoid arthritis, resign myself to an inactive, sedentary lifestyle and watch the world from the sidelines.

Those who spend time with me now would probably roll their eyes at that thought because they know I am the A-type person to fight inactivity with every ounce of energy in me. From the time I was a little girl, I would drive my mother crazy doing cartwheels and walking on my hands to the dinner table. Before arthritis as a teen-ager, most of my conversations took place standing on my head or while mastering the latest and greatest tumbling pass.

Being still, although I have grown in that aspect of my spiritual life, has never been particularly easy for me physically.

Have you heard the phrase "move it or lose it?" In this society of fast food, technology and convenience upon convenience, becoming and staying active has grown more important to personal health than ever before.

News reports address frequently the skyrocketing costs of health care, reform and the emphasis on prevention. Medical tests are expensive, and treatments for diseases (some of them partially self-induced) are often even more costly and long term.

As insurance companies raise premiums and coinsurance and decrease coverage, where does this leave you and me in a world that focuses on fixing the health problem rather than possibly preventing it in the first place?

Moving more and getting inspired for our health? I hope so.

I work for a large healthcare system and am absolutely not trying to minimize the many diseases and ailments that require vast, extensive medical treatment obtained only by skilled doctors and modern medicine. Good health, though, often starts with each individual doing his part to help prevent those illnesses directly related to poor lifestyle choices, excessive weight and inactivity.

Indiana, where I was born, raised and reside, weighs in regularly as one of the Top 10 obese states and most recently ranked as one of the unhealthiest in the nation.

Almost 20 years ago, when I was a newspaper journalist at The Republic in Columbus, I reported extensively on the state of obesity and physical inactivity and their rising concern as healthcare crises.

With more emphasis these days on the importance of diet and exercise, it would fitting to assume the overall picture of public health is improving.

Yet, in May 2012, the Indianapolis Star published a front page Associated Press article headlined, "Obesity epidemic expected to worsen" with the subtitle, "42% of U.S. adults will be obese by 2030, forecast predicts." The rapid climb of obesity rates has slowed some, but too many people in my home state and across the country are still battling the bulge.

In May 2013, the American College of Sports Medicine released its findings on the fitness of America's 50 largest metropolitan areas. Indianapolis/Carmel slipped again toward the bottom of the list ranking 45th.

Not good news.

Being obese and physically inactive are somewhat linked to a host of illnesses from diabetes to heart disease. Extra weight around the middle also puts pressure on the joints and can overall decrease one's mobility and quality of life.

As people age, movement becomes even more critical to maintain or reduce weight and to stay mobile and flexible. It increases functionality and physical fitness so individuals can walk with ease through superstores without becoming short of breath or suffering from knee pain.

Becoming and staying physically fit is about believing, and not giving up on, the ideal of healthiness and self-empowerment, even for people with limitations.

I have spent 32 years as a patient with a chronic illness, another 27 years in wellness as a professional group fitness instructor and over 15 years as an assistant in the medical field for two physician practices. All of those roles greatly differ, but they have taught me one very basic but valuable lesson in regards to personal health: the importance of taking care of yourself.

No one can do that for you or for me.

I eagerly anticipate the day when newspaper articles and government studies tout the glowing health report of America and Indiana.

It pains me to see the obesity stats and to read, yet again, how youths and adults have become even more sedentary. Isn't it time to move past this chronic state once and for all and to motivate for our health?

Enter you, by taking a leap of faith toward physical fitness and by pledging to improve your well-being.

Your joints and your waist will thank you. And if you maneuver into your skinny pants in the process, more power to you.

Getting inspired for your health is about taking charge of your personal habits to live a better lifestyle and moving more frequently for increased functionality. I know you can do it.

Chapter Two
A NEW YOU

Inspiring newcomers

Every year, new members join the gym in January, stay active for a couple of months or weeks or days, then quit by spring.

A year later, the same vicious start-stop cycle resumes all over again.

I love the New Year's Resolution exercisers. They bring a fresh spirit and enthusiasm to the gym that sometimes dwindles as my participants have spent the whole year or many years (thanks, ladies) with me.

The newcomers motivate by all of the overeating, drinking and lack of physical activity during the holidays and have faith the next year will be better and healthier.

Cheers to a New Year and a new attitude toward wellness no matter what season of life or year you find yourself reading this book. Most people, including myself, have high hopes for some healthy change to be made in their lives come January 1.

I always wonder what happens to these folks from March through December. They seem so enthused in the beginning, but one little shift in schedule—children's sports, spring break, warm weather—takes them away from their good habits and back to their old wellness rut.

On the right path

In my years of teaching fitness classes, I have noticed two things about individual habits toward exercise: more people are staying active year round, and at the same time, the ones who quit after starting a new exercise routine tend to give up more easily and quickly than ever before.

An adjustment in one's mindset toward the benefit of exercise will make this time around different for those exercise enthusiasts hanging up their athletic shoes a little too soon.

Every January, usually starting the first weekend after the New Year, the newspaper is filled with advertisements of workout clothes and equipment—anything a consumer would want to start exercising. An easy target, this fitness buff almost always purchases more workout shoes to add to an already abundant and overflowing collection.

How many times have you purchased a piece of fitness equipment, then donated it unused to next year's garage sale?

Let me console. In the past, I have been the proud owner of an exercise bike, hula hoop, stair stepper, ab machines, aerobics step, weights, resistance bands, jump ropes, balls and boxes and boxes of exercise DVDs. These are all good items, except for one very important factor: I do not like to exercise at home.

No variety of home equipment in the world will change my mind on that. My exercise gadgets remain mostly unused and nicely packaged because I am a gym rat, preferring to sweat and workout with others pursuing the same passion. Home, for me, is a place to relax.

Finding fitness success

Everyone thinks differently on where, when and how to exercise most effectively. That is where mindset and the thought put into starting an exercise routine will make or break success in becoming physically fit.

After decades of hanging out in gyms, I have seen people come and go, then come back again years later in worse shape and pounds heavier than they were before they quit. As they start the process over, the response is usually the same, "I wish I hadn't quit."

It makes me appreciate and feel blessed to teach people who have stayed committed to the gym and to their health year after year, despite schedule and life changes that occasionally get in the way of fun with fitness. Instead of looking at exercise as something they have to do, they view it as something they can do to take charge of their well-being.

Week after week and year after year, I see my class participants adjust their schedules and commitments accordingly to make at least some time for exercise.

As our society ages, becomes sicker and more obese, focusing on good health has become more important than ever. I feel fortunate to be healthy, despite having a chronic, degenerative illness. I thank God every day for the ability to move freely, walk wherever I want to walk and to lift things I never thought I could lift.

Becoming healthier begins as simply as giving up drive through windows and TV remote controls. The next time you go to the store, park in the most distant spot from the building instead of the closest or walk that extra lap around the aisles. Every bit of movement and mindfulness counts in this ongoing pursuit of healthiness.

Planning and preparation

Camp on these questions, please.

How much time do you have to exercise?

Do you have 30 minutes twice a week, 15 minutes at lunchtime five days a week, or one hour on Saturdays? Be conservative and realistic. You can always add more time.

Do you prefer to exercise at home, outside, at the gym or some other place?

This will directly relate to what types of exercises you will do, your environment and your resources. Do you have space at home to effectively work up a sweat?

How much money can you invest in this health initiative?

Can you budget for a gym membership or some training sessions if that is your preference or purchase home equipment to get you started? Remember, everyone is different, and home exercise is very effective for many people.

Do you need childcare?

Gyms have really ramped up their childcare services with the growing number of moms and dads working out. Check out their times and fees to ensure they fit within your budget and schedule.

Do you want to involve your children or spouse?

I see parents in our local parks playing Ultimate Frisbee with their kids, riding bikes on the trails or just running behind a stroller carrying their sleeping child (I don't know how they do that!).

My spouse and I usually work out separately, but occasionally we come together for a heated match of racquetball. This is something we considered when we joined the Parks Department together. The

YMCA and other family friendly facilities make it easy to get fit as a group.

Do you need the buddy system or prefer to exercise alone?

A lot of fitness books promote partners in working out, but I am going to tread cautiously here. The buddy system works well when there are safety-health considerations in exercising alone or if you have a partner who will motivate you and you inspire them. However, I have seen workout partners do a little (unintentional) sabotaging of the workout relationship. You know the type, talking you into going for ice cream instead of going to the gym. The key here is to let your inspiration guide you toward better health. Eventually, you may be the role model who motivates someone else.

AM or PM?

This one is easy. Are you rushing out the door with no time to spare in the morning and lying on the couch every evening watching television or are you an early riser with enough time to do a few sit ups or take a brisk walk before the day's activities begin? Pick your timeframe.

Do you need a scheduled time or day-by-day flexibility?

If your work or home routine varies daily, it will be beneficial to build some flexibility into your fitness plan, too. If you operate on a tight schedule, think about what times are best to incorporate exercise into your already planned day.

Do you want personal attention or group interaction?

Fitness facilities are filled with personal trainers and aerobics classes ready to get you in shape. What is your preference and interest? Many aerobics classes and leagues are free to join.

Competitive or non-competitive?

Do you have a goal such as running or walking a community mini-marathon or playing on a racquetball league, or are you content just getting in shape for yourself? I have seen many individuals truly motivate by participating in large, community fitness events.

Do you have limitations and what are they—knees, shoulders, neck, etc.?

I have worked out with rheumatoid arthritis for 32 years and have been injured once playing tennis. However, I have pushed myself too hard many times in the name of physical fitness.

Everyone, healthy or unhealthy, should seek a doctor's approval before beginning any exercise routine. Physical therapists, personal trainers and aerobics instructors can offer good advice for people with limitations. Yet, if you are working out alone or in a group setting with many faces in the crowd, it is crucial to pay attention to your body and to have some understanding of what you should and should not do.

Enjoying exercise

I know what you are thinking: it is way more fun to jump in full force and pound the pavement, right?

Weighing these considerations thoughtfully, though, will make all of the difference when the reality of crazy schedules and lives do not mesh with your enthusiasm toward starting a healthier routine.

Before closing this chapter on the beginning of a fresh, new you, let us reflect on the greatest exercise question that if left unanswered will absolutely break this healthy journey.

What kind of exercise do you like?

Do not say "none" because I know there is something out there that will inspire you to move. Is it dance, walking, swimming, hula hooping, skating, bicycling, boxing, yoga, weight training, martial arts? In modern fitness, the rules are minimal in what you can do to get your heart pumping and muscles working.

I recently attended an aerobics convention in Chicago where I spent two hours doing the Flirty Girl dance. As I shook and shimmied my way across the aerobics floor, I realized this might look prettier if I was 20 years younger, but it was fun trying something different. The classes I attended there ranged from Aqua Zumba to intense Tai Chi to a mini trampoline workout.

The combinations are limitless when developing a fitness routine. Take a few minutes now to list the exercises you have wanted or are willing to try. Remember, this is about envisioning a better you, so no need to get bogged down with too many limitations or restrictions just yet. A vast list with the potential for modification will help in future chapters to develop a fitness program suited for you.

Creating and maintaining a healthy lifestyle requires dedication and discipline. It takes work and willingness to make fitness a priority when other less healthy and more convenient choices sometimes appear so much more appealing. The goal here is balance—to work a little harder for your health so you can enjoy all of the people and things around you and to also enjoy yourself for many years to come.

Sorting through all of these important questions will go a long way in turning a fleeting desire toward healthiness into a detailed plan of becoming more active. A better, more fabulous you is well worth the time and effort. Eventually, you may be the individual encouraging all of those New Year's Resolution exercisers to stick with their good habits.

Chapter Three
FALL FOR EXERCISE

Why exercise?

In my years in the fitness industry, I have had many skeptics, non-exercisers, friends who think this passion of mine is insane ask me, "why?"

The more sedentary one becomes, the more effort it takes to gain back what is lost from physical inactivity. Exercise is crucial for endurance, strength, flexibility and balance. All four come up short when individuals live sedentary lives, which can also lead to shortness of breath upon exertion, falls and pulled muscles at even the slightest awkward move.

With my diagnosis of RA, many days I could barely get out of bed or walk across the room without hurting. My muscles were weakened, and bending to get into the bathtub for some heat relief was a huge chore.

Even after a brief period of being sedentary at age 14 due to lack of control of my illness, my endurance had decreased, strength had been zapped, balance lost and flexibility almost nonexistent compared to my pre-disease days of being a gymnast and athlete.

The summer after my diagnosis, I spent months re-conditioning myself so I could try out for the ninth-grade cheerleading squad that fall. Doing cheers and flips had once been so easy. After five months of a sedentary life, though, I could barely bend to the ground to try the splits.

My jumps (once high and effortless) were sloppy, low and painful. It took all summer to come somewhat close to re-gaining the strength, endurance and flexibility I had before RA.

Move it or lose it

Working in two very different physician practices, one specialty and one family medicine, has made me painfully aware of the state of people's health and has strengthened my desire to help more individuals get into the best shape of their lives.

The effects of excessive physical inactivity are clear. It is more difficult to travel from the parking lot to the grocery store (loss of endurance), to pick up a grandchild or run the vacuum (loss of strength), to recover when sliding on the ice (loss of balance), and to bend over and pick up something off the floor (loss of flexibility).

The less frequently individuals push themselves to move, the more abundantly this cycle continues. The effort involved in doing daily tasks and chores becomes daunting. Convenience and sedentary ways take over.

Before people realize it, they are choosing the closest parking space to avoid walking any distance, using the drive-through window instead of walking inside, and buying a riding lawn mower instead of pushing it for some extra daily activity.

We have already discussed changing mindset about exercise. Can thoughts about conveniences (at least some of the time) also be altered to slowly increase daily activity?

A few years ago, there was a push to mimic other international mobile lifestyles and walk 10,000 steps a day. Then came a more user-friendly version of that walking campaign that promoted increasing steps by 2,000 (about 1 mile) each day.

With a little planning, it is easy to incorporate some extra steps and activity into your life. Try one (or all) of these this week and see how you feel.

- Park the greatest distance from the mall
- Take the steps instead of the elevator (start small with one way if you need to)
- Walk to the mailbox, then continue around the block
- If you have easy access, ride your bike or walk to a restaurant, library, etc.
- Go to the park, and walk your dog
- Walk laps around your workplace before starting the day or at lunch

This last tip is my secret weapon toward health. I work out at the gym about three nights a week, but most days you will find me walking circles around my office building at lunchtime. Four times around the parking lot is about one mile. It takes 15-20 minutes to add that extra activity to my day.

Sometimes I walk slowly and multi-task by making phone calls. Sometimes I walk faster to increase my heart rate and endurance. Whatever the pace, it is nice to know I am making strides toward a healthier future. That little walk also gives me a few extra hours of energy to what otherwise might become a sluggish afternoon.

Endurance

Endurance is the ability to sustain an activity level. This is increased primarily with cardiovascular exercise such as walking, biking or swimming. Aerobic exercise means movement that increases your rate of breathing.

Most health organizations, on average, recommend accumulating 30 minutes of physical activity most days of the week.

When I have given talks on exercise in the past and have mentioned the guidelines, I immediately see people cringe with the thought of that much activity. Thirty minutes is a huge amount of time for some individuals, especially when freshly awakening from a sedentary lifestyle.

A goal to keep in mind is to increase your daily exercise in very small increments. Anything you do is better than nothing. So, dust off the exercise bike, and ride for a few minutes. Grab your kids, and bike or walk through the neighborhood.

Getting started is the most difficult yet important step. Even five minutes of movement is an achievement worth celebrating.

Building endurance has become essential in these days of supersized grocery stores, medical centers and parking lots. It takes a lot more steps to get in and out of facilities, and often fewer benches are available to rest.

In my years of teaching fitness classes, I have found cardiovascular activity to be a lifesaver for the mind and body. I have also found that adding more steps into the day is the easiest and most convenient way to make a big difference in one's health.

Strength

Cardiovascular activity is for lung and heart health and can also strengthen the muscles in your extremities, depending upon the exercise. When we talk about strength training, though, emphasis is mostly on resistance and weights.

The health benefits of adding moderate strengthening exercises to fitness routines include enhancing joint stability from surrounding muscles and building stronger muscles and bones.

Strength training can also help in endurance activities by making you stronger and by aiding in weight control through increasing your metabolism. Studies show resistance, along with other forms of exercise, can improve blood glucose and ease joint pain.

It may seem crazy, but when my knees hurt, I find relief in working my quadriceps (thigh) muscles at the gym through the leg extension machine or with squats. Sometimes, the first two or three are painful. Then the aching typically subsides, and I feel strength from the workout.

Strength has become increasingly important to me as I have aged. I want to continue lifting all of the things I can lift now and to bend to the floor as long as possible.

I lift weights regularly through machines and free weights. I often alter heavier and lighter resistance with fewer and greater repetitions (more reps with lighter weights, less reps with a heavier load).

A great concern of mine now with my RA is grip strength because I am constantly dropping cups, jars, etc. Many hand strengthening exercises are available. The one I find easiest and most helpful is tightening a grip and then releasing it to the fullest extension. That minimal amount of movement is beneficial for range of motion and strength of the hands and fingers.

Balance

The popularity of Tai Chi, Yoga and Pilates has generated a renewed interest in balance and flexibility, which are equally important as we age. People become frail and stiff from inactivity, which can lead to weakness, falls and pulled muscles. It is beneficial to work on balance and flexibility in a controlled setting (at home or with a trainer or physical therapist) so these principles can then be applied in daily activities.

The balance beam was my best event as a competitive child gymnast. Flip after flip, turn after turn, the moves, even on that narrow platform, seemed easy. Thirty-five years later, my balance has decreased significantly. Sometimes I can barely raise one foot off the floor without wobbling to regain control.

Hearing others struggle with the same issue, I began incorporating more balance and flexibility activities into my mainstream aerobics classes about 12 years ago. Sometimes in kickboxing, we will hold a pose for a few seconds while balancing on one leg.

I have also worked through a whole set of moves on one side in my water aerobics class so participants can practice keeping their abs engaged for more steadiness on the single foot.

On the floor, I will have my class repeat one knee lift in a controlled movement without bringing it back to the ground. If someone has balance issues, I may have them tap the toe to the floor for more stability or alternate the lift with the other leg in a slower and controlled movement. They can also hold onto the bar while performing the exercise.

Even small doses of balance activity, such as lifting a leg off the floor for one or two seconds, can increase stability and muscle strength over time. Balance exercises engage the abdominal core, which when worked can also lead to a more steady state.

To the core

Working the core has become a large focus of fitness within the last 10-15 years. Standing abdominals, enhancing the abs with resistance and combining leg and arm movements in supersets have been added to the traditional sit up to promote more power to the center.

Let's take a minute to find your core (yes, you have one).

Stand with your feet shoulder width apart and shoulders relaxed. Engage the abdominals by lifting the rib cage and bringing in the abs. This movement resembles something like putting on a pair of jeans that are too tight. Hold that position for a few seconds while continuing to breathe normally and keeping the shoulders neutral. Release. Do it again. And again. And again.

Welcome to core exercise.

Perform this activity every day for a few minutes, and you will notice a renewed strength in your center. Combining core exercise with strength, balance and endurance activities will change your physique from sedentary to strong and offer equality in all aspects of becoming physically fit. It will also make additional abdominal exercises, introduced as you progress through your fitness regimen, seem easier.

Flexibility

I subbed a Pilates class last night and realized just a few minutes in how inflexible my body felt. It had been awhile. Lately, I have been teaching a lot of kickboxing and water aerobics and have probably slighted this very important fitness category of training for flexibility.

By the end of class, I felt elongated, had better range of motion and thought I had probably grown two inches taller. Working out in a different way reminded me again of how quickly we can lose what we do not use.

Flexibility is the lengthening and stretching of muscles, and it can have a big overall impact on your well-being by increasing range of motion and decreasing stiffness. It is the one category of fitness I am thankful has been brought to light with the yoga and Pilates crowds.

I remember as a class participant years ago sneaking out of aerobics right before the stretching segment to save time. Nowadays,

I put more and more emphasis on stretching and flexibility into my classes because of their importance.

Flexibility can be as simple as reaching high for a container on the top shelf in your kitchen or stretching to the ceiling after a night's rest. Stretches should be slow, gentle and never painful. Do not bounce. The recommended duration for individual stretches is 10-30 seconds.

Long-term results

The trainings I attend as a fitness professional have changed throughout the years. Emphasis has shifted from movement just for fun to movement for functionality, especially as people age and want to remain active into their golden years.

Remember your grandparents? How physically fit were (or are) they as time has passed? I will use my family as examples of varying degrees of healthiness.

My grandmother on my dad's side was as fit and agile as they come, living independently and actively into her 90s. My other grandmother, my mom's mom, was always slightly overweight and never much into physical fitness. A former smoker, she lived a fairly healthy life into her 80s when she eventually died from lung cancer.

The quality of life was much different for these two women who were very dear to my heart.

Active Grandma was never to be found, always out late at night with her friends and traveling across the country. She sang in her church choir, attended many community functions, drove the elderly to activities, and worked countless hours coordinating cashiers for a local thrift store almost until her passing.

My other grandmother possessed a heart of gold but was never quite as active or energetic as the other. Always there when my sister and I were kids with M and Ms and popcorn during a slumber party at her house, she had a gracious spirit, but her health deteriorated with her age.

Forever a shopper, she had difficulty walking from the parking lot to the mall without becoming short of breath or using her walker. She complained of many aches and pains. Her quality of life suffered because much of the time she just did not feel well.

The difference: One grandmother was active; the other sedentary. It is never too late to improve your health through activity.

The benefits of becoming and remaining physically fit continue to evolve as studies show how much exercise can influence individual health. Finding an overall workout that flows with endurance activities, strength, flexibility and balance will move you well on your way to improved functionality and fitness.

Chapter Four
DEVELOP A PLAN

What exercises do you like?

This is the most important question to ask when developing an exercise regimen.

I will share a few of my favorites: dancing, group fitness of all kinds (kickboxing, step, Pilates, aqua), walking, weight lifting, other resistance training such as bands or medicine balls, biking, swimming and racquetball.

Then ask yourself, how would these exercises blend into my day?

I break these activities even further into categories of ones I can do alone, with my husband or friends, and those that are best for certain seasons of the year. For instance, in the warmer Indiana months, I walk, bike and swim outside. In the colder seasons, I do more group fitness and play racquetball with my husband indoors.

I fill in the gaps with weight lifting and am always open to adding something new. A few years ago, I learned to teach cycling, something I had never really desired to do but enjoyed tremendously after that initial step out of my comfort zone.

Take a few minutes to review your list of fitness activities you like or might want to try. Add or delete if necessary, but please do not be too discerning just yet. Brainstorm activities of all types-at home or at the gym, indoor or outdoor, alone or with someone else.

What do you not like?

It is also important for new exercisers to write down what activities you have tried in the past that just did not work.

Running? The cross-trainer? You know, the ones that make five minutes of effort feel like two hours. Forcing activities that are not fun or appropriate are two of the biggest mistakes I see people make at the gym, leading to burnout, frustration, possible injuries and too easily giving up on the ultimate goal of becoming physically fit.

If there is one ideal I want you to forever keep from this book, it is the concept of not wasting time on exercises you do not or will never enjoy. There are so many options out there, explore something else.

I have seen group fitness change dramatically throughout the years, always leading to another interesting format. When I first started teaching, traditional floor exercise was popular. That followed with step aerobics, kickboxing, yoga and Pilates mind-body, boot camp and now the dance craze of Zumba and hip hop. There is always something new and fresh appealing to many personalities, interests and fitness levels.

Bring out the goods

Next, take inventory of any home fitness equipment or DVDs on hand that could offer options while working throughout the rest of this book.

Do you have an exercise ball with an accompanying DVD that is screaming to come out of the spare bedroom closet? An exercise bike that initially logged miles but has been put to rest?

As mentioned previously, I am not a home exerciser. However, as my schedule gets busier and busier, I have realized the value some pieces can have in creating a time-efficient workout, especially on days when getting to the gym seems impossible. It can also be very beneficial for people who are homebound either from their health or due to caring for someone else.

Sometimes, I will spend five minutes in the morning before work doing abdominal crunches or 15 minutes before dinner working my legs and arms with weights. I am definitely a fan of home exercise equipment if it is used for its intended purpose and not just taking up space.

In the next few weeks, sort through your home equipment and discern what will be useful in your journey toward fitness. Get rid of anything you or your family will never use because looking at it only creates anxiety of not being helpful, motivating or inspiring. Also, do not buy anything else until you listen to what your body is telling you as far as exercise. Your pocketbook will thank you.

Time crunch

How much extra time do you have? That may seem like a trick question but an important one to forever break this endless cycle of active-sedentary, active-sedentary. The number one response from my students when asked why they have not been to class in three to six months is that they do not have time.

Believe me, I get it, understand it and live it. Time is always an issue. However, if you want to live to your optimum health and feel great in the process, you will have to devote some time to becoming fit.

Remember, the total weekly recommended amount of exercise is about 150 minutes, or 30 minutes most days of the week. For a sedentary person, that may seem like a large amount of time to start.

Keep that guideline as a goal to strive for as you progress in your exercise program. Let us begin more conservatively.

People lose momentum with exercise all of the time because they overestimate how much time they have. Remember the January, gung-ho, jump right in approach?

They start out with a bang, going to the gym five days a week, then realize they cannot maintain that schedule. They drop to three days, then two days, then one day, then none. Exercise no longer fits into their hectic lives.

Think about your schedule, and write down times now you can legitimately work exercise into your daily routine. Be thoughtful, specific and think long-term. I want a routine realistic enough you could still be doing it in 10 years.

For example, can you commit to 30 minutes Tuesdays and Thursdays from 6-6:30 PM? Twenty minutes Monday through Friday from 7-7:20 AM, 10 minutes every day at lunchtime or one hour Saturday morning from 8-9?

This schedule may not meet the recommended fitness guidelines, but it is a great start toward better health. The good news is that every little bit of effort counts, and more exercise can always be added later.

A tale of twos

Some people prefer to use the buddy system when working out. If you think you may want a workout partner or need one for safety-medical concerns, I would like for you to write down names of potential prospects. But, please, listen to my story first.

A few years back, a neighbor friend asked me to walk with her at 4:30 AM before work. At the time, I was teaching aerobics classes at night and not too interested in adding more physical fitness to my day. However, she was friend, so instead of saying, "no, thank you for asking" as I should have done, you can probably guess my response: "I would love to."

The first week turned out well, even though I am not an early morning exerciser and would rather have been in bed until at least 5:30. But by week two, I was losing interest. It seemed darker, colder and more painful to get up that early.

One rainy morning, my friend stopped by the house with her rain gear on and umbrella in hand-still ready to walk. I was feeling a lot less inspired, so I cancelled on her.

The best news came that weekend when she decided I was too unmotivated to continue exercising with her and ended our morning workout partnership (thank you).

Though my neighbor and I continued to walk on weekends, the problem with this morning weekday ritual was that we were not on the same page. I was sabotaging her fitness routine because I had my own schedule going at night. Thankfully, she realized I was unhelpful toward her enthusiasm and motivation.

She continued gaining her own fitness ground-solo.

Before asking a friend to join you on this fitness venture, think first about whether you really need a partner and if it will benefit both of your progress.

I am all for fitness buddies if they work well. But sometimes the best approach, especially if you are battling your own schedule and commitment issues, is to keep yourself inspired and motivated. You can always use that energy to motivate someone else later.

Shopping list

Earlier in this chapter, I mentioned not spending one more cent on home exercise equipment. However, there are three items I would like for you to purchase (or find at home) before proceeding.

We will start now increasing water consumption, so buy a colorful, inspiring water bottle to hold all of that fluid. The recommendation is 64 ounces a day, which I admit to struggling with myself. Drink up as often as you can, but especially before, during and after exercise.

The second purchase is some loose-fitting workout clothes of your choice. They can be inexpensive, but buy something that brings you joy and looks good. There are many colors and athletic fabrics in which to choose. Wearing something fun will increase your motivation.

Thirdly, and most importantly, purchase athletic shoes. Retail store shelves are packed with many varieties. They vary greatly in comfort and fit, so try on many pairs to find which one works best.

I have purchased almost every brand throughout the years and have a loyalty to each one for different reasons—the best dance shoe, the most stylish, the most comfortable, the most durable or having the best tread. I have also found that some of the less expensive shoes are sometimes as comfortable as the name brand.

Look for width, cushioning, support and what feels good on your feet. As a rule, I have discovered if they are not comfortable in the store, they are typically not comfortable later.

It is also extremely important to note that shoes most likely will not last as long as you think they should. You can extend their life by rotating pairs.

Worn out shoes, and also wearing the wrong type or size, can lead to shin splints, knee, ankle and hip problems. Replace them regularly. I buy a new pair about every three months, depending upon their use. If you think about walking toward a lifetime of fitness, that is a lot of shoes to purchase, so find the brand and type that works well for you.

When I hear of exercisers complaining of shin splints or knee pain, my first instinct is to check their shoes. Many times they look almost new on top but are worn just enough to cause injuries upon exercise impact. Switching to another pair can often lead to more miles of physical fitness.

Fit for life

As I celebrated my 46th birthday this year, I thought about the many things that are not very endearing as we grow older. Wrinkles from too much sun, memory that seems to be fading fast, clothes that are no longer age or body-appropriate and most importantly, the never ending battle to cover gray hair.

The one thing I feel so thankful for, though, is my ability to still exercise and stay active with age. Working in the fitness industry for so many years has been fulfilling and fun because the business is ever-evolving. I can always find varied approaches to old exercises and new workouts to try.

I especially admire all of the long-time fitness gurus on videos and television who continue to inspire people for their health and wellness.

It is never too late to start or restart a fitness routine. That effort begins now with discipline, planning and motivation in creating a regimen that works for you.

Chapter Five

TAKE PRECAUTION

Scenery change

Twenty seven years ago, when I first began teaching aerobics, most people joining the health club were healthy.

We pumped up our heart rates, got our blood flowing and joints moving—not worrying so much about injuries, cardiac issues, knee replacements, or falling blood sugars. Fast forward to now when more healthcare providers are writing exercise prescriptions for wellness and rehabilitation, and gyms have exploded with members entering unknown territory of physical fitness.

The landscape of the health club has changed drastically, which brings unique challenges along with the rewards for people exercising their way to better shape.

The challenge is that issues can sometimes arise when individuals transition from controlled and supervised medical care-rehab facilities to the mostly unsupervised, trendy and fast-paced fitness world. It is imperative to be smart about exercises and to always do what is comfortable and appropriate for every condition.

The rewards for new fitness buffs are clear. Many individuals can benefit greatly from adding exercise to their regular routines as far as functionality, strength and endurance. It is crucial, though, for people moving into fitness to know their body, health condition and limitations and to never be afraid to ask questions or to ask for assistance when needed.

These thoughts came to mind a few years ago when I walked into the gym in my normal routine to teach, and the picture of health I had once remembered seemed different.

To my left was an older woman on oxygen walking on the treadmill. To my right was another woman lifting weights while wearing a knee brace. In the pool area, another member, who had been absent for a while, walked lap after lap slowly in the water. She had been out for heart surgery and was continuing rehab.

Not all people at the health club are healthy these days. In fact, many members, coping with a host of illnesses, are signing on at gyms at the urging of their doctors to try a wellness approach to their continuum of care.

The idea of using physical activity as a form of preventative or continued therapy has altered the scope of what we do as fitness professionals. It has changed how we prepare programs to accommodate the masses of people with varying health concerns who share a common goal of becoming more physically fit and healthy.

Movement remedy

Traditional medicine has placed more emphasis in the last several years for patients to become a partner in their healthcare. Often times that effort starts simply with an improved diet and more exercise.

Healthcare facilities and patients are getting on board with what established disease foundations have been touting for years about the benefits of exercise.

The Arthritis Foundation has publicized its motion campaign to get the arthritis world moving more and weighing less.

The American Heart Association's website boasts a wealth of information on how exercise reduces the risk of heart disease and stroke, improves mood, offers more energy and helps people sleep more soundly.

Across the healthcare, corporate and community spectrum, efforts are being made to lead people toward healthier ways. More walking and biking paths have been added in communities across the United States. Subsidized programs offer low-cost fitness classes and recreation center memberships for seniors and other individuals. Employers promote health insurance incentives for workers taking the wellness track toward better health.

My co-workers, at the urging of one of our family physicians, participated some time back in a program to increase steps by 2,000 a day. Pedometers are still worn frequently among some employees, thanks to that initiative, and patients still remember our little friendly competition of who could become the most fit.

It is a common theory that healthcare, with its increasing expenses and decreasing insurance reimbursements, might not be in the state it is in if even more people would make a better effort to take care of themselves. Though studies repeatedly show the benefits of physical activity, only some individuals truly take that information to heart and get inspired for their health.

If there is one point I want to drive home, hammer, hit the nail on the head with this book, it is that every person can make a huge difference in his or her health for better or for worse. Choosing the better may not always be the easiest or the most convenient, but it is the best option when it comes to your longevity, well-being and functionality.

Get the green light

Everyone needs a physician's approval before beginning an exercise routine, so if you have not already done so, visit your healthcare provider for the green light on exercises appropriate for your condition. I cannot emphasize enough the importance of knowing how your body will react to exercise, especially if you have health limitations or are on medications to regulate conditions such as asthma, hypertension, arthritis and diabetes—to name a few.

These are some of the most common conditions that can be both positively affected by exercise and adversely affected, depending upon one's approach to fitness and understanding of the illness. Knowing the potential obstacles, required preparation, need for modification and realizing when to speak up will help when you discover a rough patch on your road to wellness.

At the beginning of every year, I remind my students to bring their inhalers with them to class if they have asthma and to eat something small before working out to avoid a sugar crash. Addressing all health concerns at every class is not something I practice regularly because I want to keep things fun, light and flowing well. I have gained much respect, though, for participants who know their limitations, yet do what they can to get fit and come to class prepared.

If someone in my class has an asthma attack, I want an inhaler to be on site. It is a hindrance to have the treatment 1,000 feet away and secured in a gym locker. It is also important for asthmatics to know how swimming pool chemicals will affect their breathing if a water workout is their exercise of choice.

Always speak up if doors need to be opened for increased ventilation in the pool area due to chemical levels. This is an easy fix and has helped many individuals with asthma in my aerobics classes stay active for years.

Being proactive with health conditions will alleviate a lot of concerns and anxieties about exercising safely.

Many people take medications to decrease their blood pressure or to slow their heart rate, and these drugs can affect how you feel in exercise. Inverted moves that lower the head toward the floor (as in some yoga poses) can cause a more significant drop in blood pressure and heart rate, promoting dizziness. The same move can also increase pressure on the eyes for individuals with glaucoma.

Sometimes these moves just need to be avoided and replaced with a safer option. If you are unsure how to modify a move or what to replace it with, always ask a qualified fitness professional for a better alternative, even if that means interrupting class.

I would rather have someone speak up with a question than to wonder if the move is appropriate for them or remain unsure about a more suitable exercise.

In strength training (if determined appropriate for your condition), it is important to hold the weight securely so it does not get away from you but to avoid gripping so tightly as to increase the blood pressure. Also, continue to breathe normally or count your reps.

Dizziness and loss of balance are often concerns as we age. Be careful of switching directions too quickly and participating in some of the faster dance moves. Any type of turn or spin is not a good option for individuals with balance issues, as it is easy to lose stability and fall. Exercising the option to remain forward during the movement will help prevent those problems.

Precautions also need to be taken for people with arthritis or any other musculoskeletal issues. Previously, I wrote about overdoing it as a cheerleader at the basketball tournament with my onset of rheumatoid arthritis.

The greatest lesson to take from my behavior that particular day is to ensure your disease, no matter what the ailment, is well controlled before moving forward with exercise.

As I climbed to the top of the cheerleading pyramids, I made a crucial mistake that Saturday of allowing too much body weight and awkward extension of my wrists. Then jumping from the pyramids, I leaped from an unsafe distance with unsupportive shoes for my condition and ultimately put too much pressure on my knees and ankles.

These days, I am constantly modifying dance moves that promote too much torque of the knee and yoga and Pilates poses that bear too much weight on the wrists or flexion of the knees.

I am a big fan of combining movements for supersets in many of my fitness classes but am mindful that some combinations are more effective simplified and broken down for people with arthritis as to concentrate on form and alignment.

I am also a big supporter of hand exercises, always greatly emphasizing extension of the fingers (opening up) after flexing (closing) movements because arthritic hands, including mine, often tend to be more naturally flexed.

Easy does it

I have never felt as if the no pain no gain approach is an effective way to venture into fitness. Working out appropriately in regards to time and intensity is often a matter of trial and error.

Take the easy-does-it approach for the first few workout sessions, and always err on the side of caution if you are unsure about your stamina or abilities. Pay close attention to how you feel during exercise and also the next day because your body will help guide on what and what not to do.

If I am having an arthritis flare in my left wrist, but the right one is OK, I may lift my usual weight on the right side, then either not do any on the left side or decrease the weight enough to adjust to my pain that day.

I sprained my right ankle many years ago as a kid on the gymnastics team. The ankle still gives me fits at times even today. My students will sometimes see me hopping on the left foot for more intensity, then slowing down to a light step on the right to accommodate the old injury.

It is extremely important when exercising with a health condition to monitor how you feel every day with every move.

In the past seven years or so, I have seen an influx of the diabetic patient coming into my classes. I am particularly proud of this group of exercisers because of the prevalence of Type 2 diabetes in our society.

Each of those individuals can make a significant difference in his health by improving eating habits and rethinking sedentary ways. Consider exercise, but first gain some insight from a physician about how activity will affect sugars and the way you feel.

It is important for diabetics to check sugars before, during and after exercise, at least initially, and to carry a small snack since low blood sugar can occur during activity. Even non-diabetics may notice some fluctuation in the way they feel with exercise (sometimes sugar related), so this tip can be helpful for many people.

I tend to have low blood sugar and sometimes feel that crash after exercising, especially if I do not follow my own advice and eat a little something before class to avoid shakiness. I have had other participants, especially in morning classes, feel poorly mid-way through class because they did not eat enough beforehand. Thinking and planning ahead will help alleviate potential problems like this.

Know your limits

Of all eight chapters in this book, this one on taking precautions was by far the most difficult to write because of the ever-changing health challenges in relation to the ever-changing fitness workouts.

It is so important to embrace your limits, particularly when beginning a new exercise routine. As you get into better shape, some limitations may pass, but never plow through them at the start.

It is equally critical to inform the workout facility, your instructor or trainer on specific health considerations that need to be factored into your fitness routine.

In exercise, you are pushing your heart rate to a target level, causing you to sweat, huff and puff and putting resistance on your joints that is much different than your once sedentary ways. Wearing a medical ID tag, with any illness, is beneficial so someone can have basic information on your condition if they need to help in an emergency.

Always rest when needed, especially if next-day soreness is an issue. And always keep in mind the important warning signs that indicate you should stop exercising immediately and seek assistance: chest pressure, dizziness, nausea, an unusually severe pain and shortness of breath.

The goal is to continue exercise forever, so take precaution up front by engaging your health provider in your journey and by reading on your specific health condition and how it will affect your routine. You will find much more long-term success, and that is an extra boost to your health.

Chapter Six

MOVE IT NOW, PLEASE

The first step

Did you think we would get here? All of this planning, preparation and thinking, and now we are ready to move.

Get out that new exercise outfit and shoes or pull out the one tucked in your drawer that has been screaming to be used, and let us begin.

Grab your water bottle, too, and drink up-before, during and after exercise. Consume more every day until it becomes a craving. A tip I find helpful is to have water with every meal, especially when eating out, to squeeze more in and save calories.

Earlier in this book, we addressed all of the important questions about different considerations for exercise, favorite exercises, the indoor-outdoor dilemma, and pinpointing a time in your schedule that realistically could work forever. Get your notes because it is time to put all of these thoughts into action.

First, establish your exercise time frame. Did you decide on 15 minutes at lunchtime, 30 minutes Tuesday and Thursday AM or PM, one hour Saturday or some other variation? Time is a critical factor in creating a routine that will work for you both short-term and long-term.

Time restraint

The best approach if you are time challenged—allowing only 15-30 minute increments—is to keep the routine simple with limited equipment. It is easy to waste precious time taking out gadgets, setting them up and putting them back. Just move.

I first recommend walking because it can be done almost anywhere and without changing clothes if necessary.

If you have 15 minutes at lunchtime, I want you to bring athletic shoes to work and walk on your lunch hour, either indoor or outdoor. Once this becomes a habit, purchase a pedometer and clock your steps. The calculating of steps will provide inspiration to go a greater distance each day.

Can you eventually add five more minutes? Or can you spend another 10-15 minutes after work before going home to children, spouses, dinner and laundry, logging some extra mileage?

Repeat this as often as you can until it becomes something you look forward to doing. Change your route for variety. Enlist (or drag) a coworker to come with you occasionally. Bring your MP3 player and catch up on the latest music you never have time to listen to.

When the weather takes a turn for the worse, walk inside and add staircases to your routine. You can also pump your arms for more endurance.

If walking doesn't seem like a good choice, try some yoga or Pilates moves in a quiet room in your office. Simply view a short DVD at home at another time, write down two or three moves, then incorporate them into your lunchtime workout routine. Exercise books are also helpful in displaying a few moves that can be done in a time crunch.

Chair exercises can be easily and often inconspicuously accomplished at work. Stand up from your chair and sit down 10 times. While sitting, alternate knee lifts and add some arm movements pushing forward. Change the knee lifts to low kicks and pump your arms by your side.

Always keep the core engaged for back support, and save a few minutes at the end for some deep breaths to cool down and light stretches. End by standing up and reaching tall to the ceiling or opening the arms wide.

Whatever it takes to keep you moving, just do it. When time allows, and you are able to do more, follow the next section.

Allowing more time

More flexibility definitely exists with a 30-minute workout session than with 15-minute increments. This is a good opportunity to walk for 20 minutes (starting slower to warm up, then steadily increasing the pace).

The type of warm up before exercise has been debated throughout the years. In general, the rule is to warm up (not necessarily stretch) the muscles you will eventually be working, especially the heart.

When exercising in these 15-30 minute intervals, it is best to warm up the heart by taking some deep breaths (arms reaching up on the inhale and lowering on the exhale) and by walking slowly at first, then steadily increasing that pace. The leg muscles will also warm up with the slower walk. Stretching can be done at the end of the workout.

After walking for 20 minutes, spend the next five minutes doing some sort of toning (with limited equipment because of time)-squats for legs, lifting light hand weights for arms or some abdominal exercises, either on the floor (think crunches) or standing.

For standing abdominals, position yourself like a golfer, clasping hands together in front of you, abdominals engaged and pretend to slowly raise the golf club and swing. Keep the movement controlled. Add a weight or golf club for more resistance.

For floor crunches, lie on your back, knees bent, abs engaged, and lightly put fingertips behind your head. Lift, but maintain a neutral position between your chin and your chest, keeping elbows back slightly and always remembering to breathe. It is easy to hold your breath in this position, so counting on the upward movement is an excellent way to force air.

The last five minutes will be devoted to cooling down and light stretching. Take some deep breaths to lower the heart rate. Reach your arms wide and open up the chest, a great stretch after sitting at the computer all day. To stretch the legs, rest hands at the hip bone, extend one leg in front with heel down (toe up), and bend forward slightly at the hip (chest lifted and back straight). Switch sides.

As you progress into heavier conditioning, the warm up will change somewhat depending upon the activity and may include warming up of the back and hip flexors. For now, let us keep it simple.

Once you have established a 30-minute routine several times a week and have become comfortable with your choice of activities, pull out your expansive list of exercises you would like to try and add something new, such as riding your bike or doing an exercise video. Plenty of good DVDs are on the market that will give you an overall workout with a qualified instructor.

Remember the guidelines of accumulating 30 minutes of exercise most days of the week? Adding more of those half-hour segments to each week will enhance your fitness level more rapidly. If, at some point, you can increase to 45 minutes, just add small amounts of time to your endurance, strength and stretching segments.

One hour workout

For individuals who have one hour on any day to work out, I would initially break it into intervals like this: Ten minute warm up (some deep breaths and light walk), followed by 20 minutes of brisk walking (cardio), followed by 15 minutes of leg, arm and abdominal toning (squats, light weight lifting, standing or floor abs), and finishing with 15 minutes of cooling down (walk in place, deep breaths) and stretching. End of workout stretching will be more important in this scenario because of the increased length of the workout.

This is a tentative schedule because of the time flexibility to adjust the workout however you feel that day. Never feel obligated to one exact routine. Customizing a workout to your enthusiasm and energy level for the moment will make the routine forever-changing, which helps tremendously in avoiding plateaus.

You can also add more equipment in a one-hour workout routine. For variation, jump rope, swim, watch a DVD or ride your bike instead of walking. Do some jumping jacks for endurance alternating with intervals of weight training. Anything goes. Mix it up as much as possible for the best training effect and so this will be a fun habit and not something you dread doing.

A good fit

Any exercise is time well spent and will move you farther along to where you want to be physically.

A lot of interesting and sometimes conflicting reading is available on exercise. For beginners, just trying to get into the habit, I advise this:

- Keep it simple, especially if time and motivation are issues. I have seen people quit exercising because they do not feel like packing their bag that day or driving 10 minutes to the gym. If something is not working for you (such as these examples), change it. Exercise at home for a few weeks where it is more time-efficient and convenient. Walk around the neighborhood, so you do not have to change your clothes (yet always wear athletic shoes).
- If you are feeling anxious because of all of the goodies you ate over the holidays or at a summertime cookout, work out. A 30 minute walk will do wonders for your mind, anxiety and energy.
- If you are feeling sluggish, unmotivated and do not feel like sticking to your established routine, make yourself do some sort of exercise for five minutes. Most of the time once started, you will continue longer.

Please do not give up on exercise because you feel time is the issue. Studies have shown that even short increments (10 minutes) can provide some health benefit, increase energy and improve mood.

Sometimes I spend two hours at the gym, and sometimes I squeeze in 10 minutes of exercise at home. Even minimal activity will keep you in the mindset of pressing onward for your health.

Exercise vs. activity

It is important to understand the difference between exercise and activity because both can be beneficial in your journey toward wellness.

At the time I started writing this book, all of my aerobics classes were cancelled because of the Thanksgiving holiday. I was sort of at a loss for what to do with my time and energy.

I cleaned the house from top to bottom because of company arriving soon. I spent hours sweeping, dusting, mopping, cleaning the refrigerator and closets. Can you tell it had been awhile?

I decorated for Christmas, dug up the last of my dying outdoor flowers, washed my car, went to the grocery store and finished my Christmas shopping-all before black Friday.

I was tired and satisfied with what I had accomplished. However, even with all of that activity, my exertion level still did not measure up to the way I felt after finally getting back to the gym for an hour of exercise the next Saturday morning.

I admit that some household chores are pretty darn strenuous. (Think gardening, cleaning out the garage, and painting). Yet, a difference exists in the exertion level between those activities and physical fitness.

Although I do not feel chores can take the place of exercise or offer the same health benefit, there is definitely some significance to adding more activity and movement, of any level, to your life.

So many ways present in our daily routines to squeeze in extra activity and exercise without being too time cumbersome.

- Stand while folding laundry
- Take the stairs
- Walk your dog instead of letting her into the yard
- Ban drive through windows forever
- Rethink the remote control

I admire a coworker friend of mine because she always wears a pedometer, clocking her steps wherever she goes and always striving to add a little more movement.

I know you can be creative, too. Just keep your mind focused away from those sedentary ways and toward your new life of activity and physical fitness. Move it now, please.

Projecting exertion

Exercise will sustain your elevated heart rate for an extended period of time leading to cardiovascular fitness, while activities typically do not. You can monitor the rising of your heart rate a couple of different ways. Two practical ways are by perceived exertion (or how you feel) and the talk test.

If you feel like you are working hard and are somewhat huffing and puffing, then your heart rate is most likely elevated. If you can tell a 30 minute story, all while working out, your exertion level could probably be increased.

The key to an effective workout is to balance the two. You should be able to talk some during exercise even if your heart rate is up, but you should not be able to continue a long conversation in order to reap the most physical benefit from your efforts.

If you have difficulty saying a few words during an exercise routine, slow things down a bit until that excessive windedness subsides. If you can speak well through the whole workout, moving at a faster pace will increase your exertion level.

One way to elevate your pulse, especially with an activity like walking, is to add various arm movements in a controlled manner such as pumping your arms or raising them up and down above your head. In fitness classes, you will see combinations of leg and arm movements for increased heart rate.

Though perceived exertion is often used to measure the intensity of a workout in the fitness industry today, wearing a heart rate monitor and knowing your target and maximum heart rate can also be beneficial. Heart rate monitors are available in many stores and on-line because of the demand for more accuracy in calculating exertion levels.

Even though it is broad, I like this manual formula to identify your estimated target heart rate. Subtract your age from 220 (this would be your age predicted maximum heart rate), multiply that number by 60 and 80 percent. The range of the two numbers would be your simplified target heart rate range.

This target heart rate formula is based on your age, but it is also important to keep in mind the medications you take, your health condition, exertion capabilities and goals established by your health provider. It is often beneficial to go by target heart rate in addition to perceived exertion in regards to your workout level for the day.

Always something new

The beauty of modern fitness is that it can be ever-changing just as our bodies and our energy levels are ever-changing. Exercising is a hobby that truly ages with you.

When I first started teaching aerobics at age 19, I instructed mostly advanced classes. That regimen worked well for many years until I started feeling fatigued from too much exercise.

I then incorporated some beginning and intermediate classes into my week and found relief from the mix in routine. These days, I teach only two classes, one advanced floor class and one aqua aerobics class, and enjoy the variety in subbing for others as much as possible.

After so many hours spent at the gym, I have learned that long-term consistency in exercise-not always time spent per session-goes a long way toward improving one's health. I have also learned the benefit and time savings of incorporating more activities into my daily routine.

At least once a week, for my mind and body, I absolutely must work out hard, get my heart rate up, and sweat off the stress of the week. The next week, I do it again but often in a different fashion.

I am always eagerly anticipating the next big fitness craze finding its way into fitness facilities, but until that time comes, incorporating more and more of what I know to be beneficial and effective in exercise keeps me moving now and hopefully for many years to come.

Chapter Seven
THE DIET DILEMMA

Diet overindulgence

America weighs heavily on diet overload. Millions of individuals diet each year, and billions of dollars are spent on weight loss products.

The ideal of losing weight through diet appears to have become a national pastime.

The issue? Our society continues to grow heavier and more sedentary, as studies report. Those facts bring to debate the role obsession with scales and food consumption really plays in the quest for healthiness.

I have seen people lose weight through various diets and keep the pounds off. I have seen people lose weight through various diets and gain the pounds back.

I have seen people truly enjoy the latest weight loss plan and follow every step of its path. I have seen people dread the thought of watching what they eat, yet they do it again in the name of losing weight.

I have seen people nearly disrobe before getting onto the scale. I have seen people weigh on one scale, then go to another for a potentially different reading.

One little tip as we venture through this touchy subject about weight together: Throw out your scale at least for this chapter. No one needs a scale to tell them how healthy they feel.

Healthy ideal

This book has nothing to do with what diets you have tried and possibly failed, how much you weigh or how tightly your clothes fit compared to last year. It has everything to do with how much healthier you can be through physical fitness and striving to make better choices in eating and other health habits.

If there is one point I want to clear up about the pursuit of healthiness, it is that being thin and being physically fit are two totally different ideas and concepts. Just because someone is thin does not necessarily mean that person is healthy or fit. On the contrary, just because someone appears heavier does not necessarily mean that individual is unfit.

I have seen a lot of thin, young girls who struggle to finish my fitness classes. I have had older, somewhat overweight women who can do my class and another one all in the same day.

Research has indicated that waist circumference plays a role in your good health, but our society places way too much emphasis on diets and being thin.

I would much rather see a person active, functional and fit than to just be skinny.

That said, it still takes both exercise and eating better (not necessarily dieting) to create a well-rounded approach to good health and to reach and maintain optimum weight.

You will most likely never see the weight loss results you desire with exercise alone. You also will never reach the physical fitness, endurance and functionality level you would like with diet alone.

A better way

Last year, I volunteered several Saturdays at our local free health clinic offering advice on the importance of personal health. Since my expertise is in fitness, I had prepared to discuss more on exercise and less on diet choices. A dietitian was available for nutritional information.

As I conversed with patients for several hours those weeks, stories of unhealthy eating unfolded. Confession after confession of diet troubles made me very aware of the great nutritional dilemma in our society.

Plain and simple: Individuals need to eat better. Exercise is an easy and effective habit to start, but breaking these diet roadblocks is crucial to travel the narrow path of health and wellness.

Four of the five people I chatted with one morning drank a 2 liter of soda daily. One person purchased fast food for every meal and another consumed her meals from the vending machine at work.

For several of these individuals, their cholesterol, blood pressure and sugars were out of control. They had gained pound after pound throughout the years, which were even more difficult to shed as they aged and became less active. Combine their poor eating choices with sedentary lifestyles, and a health disaster erupts.

These folks definitely benefitted from some guidance about exercise that day. But when diets are filled with fats, sugars and patterns of unhealthy choices, which they too often are, even the most consistent exercisers will struggle.

Think about your food choices and eating habit weaknesses. Choose one area you struggle with most in your diet.

Just as my friends at the clinic with the excessive soda intake, I, too, struggle with drinking too many calories. I consume one regular soda daily and too many fruit juices. One habit I recently broke was putting sugar in my coffee, first switching to a substitute and now just milk.

For some individuals, their weakness is sweets; for others it is eating out. Others struggle with late night dining, portion control, fast food or boredom consumption.

Late night eating runs a close second to my sugary drink issue. I often teach aerobics after work, forcing me to eat late, and ultimately, eating too much because I have worked all day, just worked out and feel hungry.

These habits prove the challenge of doing right in regards to health sometimes does not work well with busy schedules and multiple commitments. Two options exist: Continue the unhealthy, convenient pattern of eating, or consistently make better choices that fit with hectic lives.

To accommodate for my late nights, I typically opt for a larger, more nutritionally balanced breakfast and lunch, then a much smaller and lighter dinner. I have also cut my portions by about one-third of what they used to be and realize I am still full.

Take account

What is your eating weakness? Write it down now, please.

When I learned at the clinic these individuals were consuming almost 2 liters of soda daily, I immediately asked them to cut the amount in half and replace the other half with water. They may never be able to give up soda completely but just decreasing their consumption would drastically slice caloric intake and improve their health. My goal for them was to eventually consume just one canned soda daily.

To curb a sweet tooth, I often recommend eating a miniature candy bar instead of a full size, drinking a small glass of chocolate milk, consuming a 100 calorie snack, or chewing the latest dessert gum. It is also helpful to fill up on water or something healthier before satisfying a sweet craving to avoid overeating of the unhealthy item.

For many people, fast food is a prime diet buster. These days, restaurants are forever bustling with patrons.

The best approach is to decrease the number of times eating out and to buy more healthful groceries to fix at home. If you dine out six meals a week, decrease that number to three. If you eat out three meals a day, slice that to one meal.

Most restaurants offer nutritional information on their menu items, so it is more convenient to read up and develop an eating out plan. Scheduling a dietitian consult, sometimes free through local health organizations, is a great resource to help improve eating both at home and when dining out.

Do you find yourself going to the pantry every 10 minutes to see if the selection has changed?

The best approach to boredom eating is to have some healthy items on hand that are quick and easy to grab, such as bagged carrots, nuts (instead of chips) and fruit. It is also helpful to take cues from our previous chapters and hit the pavement for a walk instead.

Exercise may ultimately take your mind off of food.

Back to the basics

Diets have become very complicated and crazy throughout the years with all of the fads, trends and weight loss promises. Getting back to the basics is a great way to simplify and rethink what individuals are putting into their bodies and why.

It is important to always ask: Am I even hungry?

Forget the scale and weight loss goals for now, and focus on the very small dietary changes that can improve one's overall eating habits. With long-term weight control, it is often the simplest adjustment that will have the most impact on health. Combining more effective, thoughtful eating with a less sedentary life may eventually turn obesity from a national epidemic to a minor ailment.

Chapter Eight
GET INSPIRED .... AGAIN

Keep going

Today is February 12, and I just finished reading a small newsletter article from a national fitness organization about apathy that hits gyms now and the remaining 10 months of the year.

Six weeks into the New Year, classes are beginning to slow down from the holiday rush, and enthusiasm toward exercise is dwindling. The article charged fitness instructors to keep participants motivated for their health, despite schedule changes and other obstacles pulling them away from their good habits.

People ask me all of the time the secret to keep going. They know I work long days at the doctor's office, go to my second job as an aerobics instructor, and write on the side.

Night after night, year after year, I head to the gym to teach my routine time slots, and sometimes, after almost three decades, I question whether I can do it one more time.

Some days I am running on adrenaline after work, ready to teach a class, lift weights and swim laps. Other days, the better choice seems to be the couch for a nap and quick dinner.

I think we all have those days when crashing at home sounds much more appealing than any form of physical exertion. I am the first to admit that occasionally, very occasionally, the best choice is to give up on exercise for the day and get some much needed rest and relaxation.

The next day, however, it is time to move it and move on and get back on track with your fitness regimen. Never let that one day become six days or six months or six years.

Staying consistent and committed are the keys to getting you in the best shape of your life and keeping you there.

When I was first diagnosed with rheumatoid arthritis, it took years to find medications that worked well and kept my disease under some sort of consistent control. I missed a lot of school and felt challenged by small tasks of walking across the room or picking up the laundry basket.

Giving in to my joints often seemed like the best and easiest option, but my stubbornness and naivety would never let that happen. I pushed through and am thankful to move more freely today.

Enduring a chronic disease has taught me a lot about myself and the importance of maintaining strength. The most enlightening fact is that I can make a huge difference in the quality of my life just by actively participating in my health.

Even these days, though my RA is well-controlled, the common aches and pains associated with aging are sometimes enough to make me forget the gym and hang up my athletic shoes. Throw in an acute illness, upper respiratory infection, headache, Lazy Day Syndrome, etc., and camping out at home looks better all of the time.

Appealing, sure, but how about getting inspired again instead?

Motivation to the end

The most effective way to keep going in this plight toward health is to change your routine as your body, interests and schedules change.

For years, I instructed as many of the most difficult classes I could possibly do in a week. That regimen worked, despite having RA, because I was young, fit and could easily maintain this rigorous workout program.

These days, I would be sore for days trying to copy that same schedule, so I teach a more appropriate level for my age and mix workouts up frequently to prevent burnout, injuries and fatigue. I am always looking for something new and exciting to motivate myself and my students.

In 2007, I certified in Zumba, which was very different at the time with its Latin music and hip-shaking moves. My latest interests are line dancing with its fun music and choreography and Tai Chi with its slower, more controlled standing movements.

The first part of this book focused on developing the right mindset for fitness, and at that stage, it is easy to be excited about exercise. The hard part now is continuing to pursue those fitness goals and maintaining momentum for years down the road.

Keep these thoughts in mind.

- Always be open to something new. If a friend invites you for a hike in the park, put on your hiking boots, and seize the moment. If the neighborhood kids are jumping rope, show them your moves, too. There is always something fun to try in the name of physical fitness.
- Move your workout from indoors to outdoors. Taking advantage of weather changes to do something different with a routine is an ideal rut-fixer. Enjoy the scenery of parks, beaches, mountains, etc. instead of the small walls of the gym.
- Stir up the mix. Some activities you may not want to do all of the time, but they could come in handy for an occasional change in workout. Think roller or ice skating (if your body allows), partners tennis, bowling, golf, Frisbee and fund raising walks, which are held year-round.
- Try a home boot camp. Ride bikes to the park, then walk the trails. Combine chores such as cleaning out the garage by enlisting everyone in the family. Race to see who can remove the most items from the garage the fastest, clean the area, then put things back nicely into place.

- Change your timing. If you are comfortable working out in the morning but could benefit from a temporary reprieve, switch your routine to nights for a couple of weeks. Or move your lunchtime weekday fitness routine to weekends. The change does not have to be permanent. A brief switch in the normal schedule may be just enough to renew your enthusiasm.

- Groove to the music. Personal electronics are sophisticated and geared to keep you motivated when working out. Redefine your playlist with new music that motivates you to move.

- Exchange land for water. Transitioning from land to water (or water to land if you are typically an aqua exerciser) is one of the best changes anyone can make to mix up the routine. Many exercises are interchangeable (slower paced in water and faster on land) and will provide a totally different workout in the new environment.

- Add more equipment. Trying something new such as resistance bands instead of free weights or large exercise balls in place of a mat will add a whole new dimension to strength training. Jump ropes and mini-trampolines can shake up endurance moves.

- Introduce lateral moves. Most exercises flow in a forward pattern such as walking. Initiating some lateral movements, such as a side step, will train the body differently.

- Find a friend. Now is an excellent time to bring a workout partner occasionally into the mix since you have mastered the self-motivation to stay fit. Because people have varied interests, choose someone different for each activity you enjoy.

Fitness remix

Varied exercise routines that are developed appropriately can offer maximum training results while decreasing the risk of injury. The principles of frequency, duration, intensity and mode of exercise are common techniques among fitness organizations to adjust exercise routines for schedules, interests, abilities and athleticism. Variables include frequency and length of the weekly workout sessions, difficulty of the routine and type of exercises performed. The interrelating of these four factors can help create a balanced program to increase continued interest and to help reduce the risk of injuries.

For instance, if you increase the intensity of your workout by kicking it up a notch, most likely the length of your session will decrease initially to accommodate for the greater difficulty. If you add another mode of exercise, the duration will also probably decrease because of the varied training on the body with the new activity.

If frequency of workout sessions is increased, intensity will often decrease to adjust to the greater time spent working out. On the contrary, if frequency of workout sessions decreases, difficulty can easily be increased to compensate for fewer days at the gym.

Gradual increases and changes in frequency, duration, difficulty and type of exercise will allow for proper progression of your workout routine to enhance your fitness strength and stamina. Once in an established workout regimen, occasional switching of these variables will keep the routine interesting and challenging. Increasing time spent working out will also move you toward the recommended guidelines for exercise.

Increased momentum

You have come a long way in this book from finding a new you to falling for exercise to staging a wellness plan. You have the knowledge to take precaution at times in setting up a routine that works well and to pay closer attention to what role foods play in regards to your health and weight.

Getting inspired again is the best place to be in this health journey because you have done it once, and it is easy to fuel the fire you first had toward fitness.

I am looking forward to teaching my class this Wednesday night and increasing our normal duration of abdominal exercises from five to 15 minutes. The next week, I will increase the intensity of our endurance segment by jumping rope.

My poor class participants never know what workout awaits them each week. Fortunately, as long-time exercisers, they are always smiling and eager to try something new.

That enthusiasm makes my small weekly commitment to them well worth the effort again and again.

I feel fortunate to have spent the greater part of my life motivating people toward better health, and I am grateful for all of the individuals in my world who have inspired me to do the same.

Getting inspired and staying motivated-that is what life-long health and wellness is all about. It is never too late to join in the fitness effort, and it is never too late to recommit to healthier ways again.

Conclusion

We're not done yet.

That is the line I often use on my exercise students with about 20 minutes remaining in class when their energy is draining and enthusiasm somewhat waning.

They usually laugh, roll their eyes and shout some words at me.

What I am really implying in these last few moments together—pushing through the sweat and fatigue—is that the best is to come.

If you have not totally figured out this health and wellness venture yet, let me reassure you the best is to come. It is your turn to wholeheartedly participate in your health now in whatever ways you feel fit your lifestyle and your needs.

After arriving home from aerobics conventions, I usually bring back notebook upon notebook of choreography ideas and exercise and nutrition tips to pass onto my classes. At first glance, it seems overwhelming and difficult to remember anything I learned from the workshops.

That may be what you are feeling now after learning the history of strides to get people moving and by realizing all of the ways exercise can benefit your health and fit into your day.

I find slowly incorporating small bits of information is a much more manageable approach than trying to do everything at once. When I return from the workshops, I often introduce only one new choreographed eight-count each month until it becomes easy for me and the individuals taking my classes.

Setting small goals may work best for you, too, as you mindfully introduce some of these fitness principles into your life. Weeding through what works now and what could work later will also help in creating a fitness routine to start as soon as possible and offer flexibility when the mix needs stirred to avoid plateau.

As we part ways, I have one more question to always ponder before introducing new exercises into your life.

Is the exercise safe and appropriate for you?

When I began writing this book, I talked myself out of writing strictly about exercise and arthritis because I have always followed a much more aggressive fitness path than what has been protocol or recommended for people with rheumatoid arthritis.

Upon my initial diagnosis of RA, I searched for any treatment possible to help me because at that time medications were only somewhat beneficial, and children were not treated very aggressively.

My first line of medicines consisted of daily mega doses of aspirin. Though I quickly climbed the medication therapy ladder, my joints remained swollen and hurt constantly, and I could feel my strength, flexibility and endurance decreasing almost daily.

I felt sort of helpless with my condition, so I turned to the one therapy I had always known and thought would continue keeping me strong and healthy, despite dealing with RA.

Exercise.

The modern medications I take now keep me mobile and moving toward a healthier way of life. Even though I can participate in most fitness regimens, I am constantly weighing whether they are safe and appropriate for my condition and age. The continued questioning of what I should and should not do has saved me throughout the years, especially as I pursued fitness outside of the traditional exercise and arthritis norm.

The key to exercising well is to do so without injuries. Safety comes with variety, modification, carefully considering whether the benefit of a particular move is worth the risk and resting when needed.

Exercise has been such an important part of my life, I would not change anything about my pursuit of fitness throughout the years or trying to get others motivated for their health. I am thankful for all of the community and company efforts—weight loss challenges, fitness classes, health fairs, etc.—that inspire people to care for themselves even more.

How healthy are we?

We're getting there. It takes everyone's discipline and dedication to help wellness in America find its glory as the center of attention, rather than the clichéd plight of unhealthiness. I will call it a MOVEment in the right direction.

About the Author

Cheryl Fiscus Jenkins was diagnosed with rheumatoid arthritis at age 14. Staying mobile and not being confined to a sedentary life is the backbone of why she is writing this book today. She has spent the past 27 years in the fitness industry, teaching aerobics classes of all levels in various health clubs throughout Indiana.

Cheryl is certified through the Aerobics and Fitness Association of America and works for AFAA as an Indiana Examiner for primary group instructor trainings. She is also certified in Keiser cycling and is trained in step aerobics, aqua, kickboxing, Pilates, hip hop, Latin dance and weight training.

Cheryl writes "MOVE" with a conversational style, stemming from her column-writing experience as a journalist. She graduated from the University of Evansville in 1990 with a bachelor's degree in communications/journalism. After graduation, she wrote for The New Albany Tribune and The Republic newspapers in Indiana, covering news, features and sports.

In the mid-1990s, she won awards for "Best In-Depth Feature Story" writing from the Indiana Associated Press and Hoosier State Press organizations.

After serving as a reporter and Features Editor for many years, Cheryl returned to school to pursue a career in healthcare. She has a certificate of medical assisting from Ivy Tech State College and has worked in the medical field since.

Cheryl began activity early as a gymnast and cheerleader. During college, she performed with the half-time dance team and was a member of Alpha Omicron Pi sorority, where she worked many philanthropic events for the Arthritis Foundation.

In her spare time, Cheryl travels and rides bikes with her husband, Matt. She also enjoys serving as Deacon of her church in Franklin, Ind., and spends time in Florida with her retired parents.

Cheryl can be reached for correspondence at moveinspiredhealth@ gmail.com.

Helpful Resources

American Diabetes Association

America's Health Rankings

American Heart Association

America on the Move

Arthritis Foundation

Centers for Disease Control and Prevention

ObesityinAmerica.org

Parks and Recreation departments

President's Council on Fitness, Sports and Nutrition

Shape Up America!

U.S. Department of Health and Human Services

Notes

Notes

Notes